SEX HEALTH AND BETTER SEX

TABLE OF CONTENTS

INTRODUCTION / MY TWO CENTS

Understanding sex is as important as living life. Sex is healthy, a good stress reliever and natural. Sex is done more mentally than physically because 75% of people who have sex don't get satisfied, or say get that perfect sex. But we're talk about that later. Sex is unpredictable even though it feels the same all the time, but it depends on your partner. Both have to be into it in order to be at peak but if one of the partner not interested, then the overall performance will flop or won't be that great. Neither one should force their partner to do anything they are not interested in because that will most likely scar the relationship. So before you fall in love and get in a relationship with someone, make sure you two agree on everything about sex. Because if you marry a person who doesn't give head and you like receiving head then you'll have problems during your relationship and may result to adultery. If you like licking ass and your partner don't agree, and then your relationship will be ass out. That's why sex is a major part of a relationship. I'm only speaking in a married perspective way. I can't promote fornication otherwise I'll be a hypocrite and everything I said can't be addressed to two people that's in love. So if you just got a sex/fuck buddy, this may not apply to you because I wrote everything to approve married relations. "Don't watch porn" if you don't know by now porn can ruin a relationship for a couple who's been married even 30 years. It has a negative influence and creates urges to cheat on your partner, besides the sex in porn is not real. 90% of people in porn don't even enjoy it, they just there for the money. So if you want to strengthen your relationship with your partner, avoid Porn at all cost. Because the moment you watch other people have sex you'll start to commit fornication consciously, then your mind starts to wonder. If you just trying to get a hard on, it only means your partner is not attractive anymore even when he/she is naked. Because if my wife says she has to watch some porn to get in the mood, I'll consider that as an insult. Dropping my Hanes should be enough for her. So if you a man and can't get and can't get a hard on or if you a woman and can't get wet, only physically changes need to be made.

NOTE: *men are born between a woman's legs and spend the rest of their lives trying to get back between them. Why? Because there's no place like home*

PREPARING FOR SEX

Would you eat a meal an hour before you play basketball or a track meet? No, right, so since sex is like aerobic exercise, it's a good idea not to eat anything before sex and most definitely not to load up on sugar as it deploys the urge to be active. Best bet is drinking ginseng, or vitamin water an hour before you get into it. It's also good to stretch out your legs and arms for better performance and blood flow. Try not to stress over anything and just think about the nakedness of your partner and what you would like to do to him or her. If you need extra help to feel the urge, try phone sex with your partner first and then when she/he walks in the door you should be more than ready. If you need to spice things up, send naughty texts back and forth all day until you two get home and finish the story. Play strip trivia- ask each other questions and whoever answers wrong has to strip off a piece of clothing. Have a lap dance. Send naked photos to each other, creating a higher desire. But this can be dangerous, I advise couples to delete pictures after it's been seen already. Record the sounds of your moans when having sex with each other, then when you two get home, play the sound on your cd player. Make your kisses more passionately. Have sex blindfold. Use food like ice pops and whip cream and blueberries. Play wrestle with no clothes on, and whoever gets pinned or tap out has to let their lover take control. Bite and nibble for 10 minutes. Slip a donut on his penis and slowly lick it off. Be careful with fantasy dress-up sex because some imaginations can create a negative desire.

NOTE: *To keep your relationship healthy, have sex daily or at least 3 times a week. If you wait too long to have sex again you can lose desire in your mate and see him/her as unattractive. Females, if you want to keep your man overdose him, make sure he's addicted to you, and be careful with that vaginal probation crap. That doesn't works, only gives a man a reason to cheat.*

PLACES TO HAVE SEX

Sometimes you want to extend your sex life somewhere else other than the bedroom. The shower is the most relaxing place to have sex. It's like getting a massage and getting an orgasm at the same time. Especially if you have back problems, while the warm water crashing against your back, you're enjoying your penetration with your partner. If you got the freak in you and want to enjoy a freaky moment, then car sex or in the back seat of your car is perfect to get all the freakiness out of you to release some stress. Don't worry; being a freak means you're healthy and sexually active. Those who are not a freak in the bed are most likely the worst lovers, and when they have an orgasm it's nothing. So be a freak and have some freak sex. I don't prefer floor sex unless you have very strong knees and back, and a soft carpet. Floor sex is the cause of many back aches and pains. So I avoid this unless I have a sleeping bag. A sleeping bag is perfect for the cold days and it keeps you and your partner close together, the experience is great but the cleaning is difficult. Kitchen counters sex, for me personally, I don't like to have sex anywhere you prepare food at. But if you want something new, go for it. Park sex; hey don't be a shame because in the historic days when there were no houses, that's when making babies took place. Parks and gardens were called homes to people B.C. So go head and give a park a chance to take your sex to exceed your limits. It's fun, beautiful and the air makes it better. But you should not do it in from of people because sex is personal and should only be seen by the only two people that are doing it. Only birds and squirrels may see you but they aren't telling anyone you know. The best time to have sex in a park is when it's fall and cool and the leaves are fallen. Another good place to have sex is the Jacuzzi. It may be difficult for a male to get an erection in the water but once he does, it's a great experience, because of the relaxation you're getting from the Jacuzzi. A paddle boat in the middle of the ocean is a dream fantasy to make love at. It's nothing but the moans and waves and water that'll make the sex 10x better. But make sure there's any sharks in the area you plan. Also roof sex is great but you and your partner can't be seen by the public, so the roof should be high enough and flat. Make sure you have a flat roof so neither you nor your partner falls off. We all heard about sex on the beach before, just make sure you have a towel to lay on your body on and go to work. It's so relaxing, it's better than a honeymoon in a hotel. You get to hear the waves sing and the birds tweet. While the sand massages your back while making love. If you fortunate enough and can own a private plane, it's calming to be stroking with your partner in the air if you get butterflies during plane rides. But it has to be a private plane with just you and your wife. It'll be a good idea to throw on some music because you don't want the guy who's flying your plane to be masturbating. Another sexual fantasy place is a cave, and if you can find a cave, go head and give it a try, but watch out for the cave monsters, public restaurants is too dirty, I won't recommend that but if you can bring your own cleansing products, it might work.

NOTE: *The best sex to have is after an argument. After cursing each other out and saying the worst things to each other, just strip your clothes off and jump in the bed and have rough sex. It may not solve the problem but it'll ease the situation and make the problems easier to solve. It's a high but*

natural.

AFTER SEX

After sex mood depends on what was the performance like or how good the sex was. If a cigarette is smoked after sex, it means the satisfaction was insufficient. The potential of the best sex possible wasn't reach and there's still stress hanging over your heads. If you fell asleep after sex or forgot the argument you was having, then that means the sex did what it was supposed to do. Now if you and your partner are still arguing and fighting and cursing each other after you two just had sex, then that means the sex was bad. Cheap sex that can't be remembered, sex that didn't intercept the mind, sex that just didn't make anything better, so you and your partner rush to put your clothes back on. She grabs a cigarette and you call your homie for a bag of weed because you two are trying to forget the moment that just happened. Cigarettes is for calming down, because women liked to be calmed down when stress. Weed is for to relax through a meditation high because men want to skip over and forget their problems. The only thing that can calm down a woman and make and make a man forget his problems is great sex that'll never forget. Sex only start off bad if both not into it or just one is into it. Most likely somebody in the relationship has to be a freak and teach his/her partner to be one as well. Freak doesn't mean whoring or being a slut, it just means you like sex, which is healthy and you are sexually active. People who aren't having sex usually have higher rates of heart attacks.

NOTE: *The only way to make sure your relationship is at the strongest peak, if you or your partner is not embarrass of each other nakedness and that you two are having great sex. If you and your partner is married and she or he still comes out the shower with a towel covering his/her body when it's just you two in the house, then that should tell you that your relationship is weak. A good relationship is confident, trusted, honest, loving and happiness. If you don't feel any one of these, then you might have to make a decision.*

MASTURBATION

For women it's not bad, it's more like an appetite but the nails on your fingers can scratch and damage the clitoris. But for men it can be used to get an erection but the consequences of masturbation is erectile dysfunction because the penis can get used to getting an erection from the hand and adopt orders from the brain telling it to only get erected from using the hand. So if the man can only get his penis hard by stroking it, he will develop sexual problems later on. Like most likely he'll lose erection during intercourse because the penis is used to being pleasured by the hand. So men try working on getting an erection only from the mind, from the look of a woman, which is only natural and tended to be. If you don't have a partner, don't be embarrassed to use a sex doll or sex toy, because 80% of women have their little secrets under their mattress. The closer you are to the real thing, the better chance your penis will recognize the real thing. Think of your penis as a password to a PC, and you keep logging in using Guest(hand), soon you'll forget your password when you try to log in on your username(partner's vagina) Well masturbation does help prevent rape and sexual abuse but you have to use it wisely.

CONDOMS

Condoms are safe but it's unnatural. But if you want to be safe you got to sacrifice 80% of the feeling. If you want 100% of the real feeling then you're going to have to take the risk of catching a STD, AIDS or even dying. It's not fair because every time a person gets into the mood for sex, first they have to think about life or death. When a man is putting on a condom, he really don't want to put it on but his conscious is stuck on an STD and a woman most of the time worries about getting pregnant more than catching something. This is why the creator created sex only for the two people that are married because fornicators transfer body fluids to another person body to another which can transfer blood. So it's best to stay monogamous with only one partner.

ORAL SEX

Unless you want to contract an incurable STD, I advise you to wash your mouth before and after you give your partner oral sex. Brushing your teeth and or using mouth wash are a good idea but hydrogen peroxide is perfect for washing away germs in your mouth. Use it if you don't want to transmit the germs in your mouth to your partner private area. And it's also a good idea to wash your vagina or penis before and after oral sex to prevent any STD.

NOTE: *There's no limit where a couple should have sex because true love have no limits or shame. Not saying that it's good to have sex in public where people could see you, but if you have public sex like in a park or train station, it should be private because sex is sacred. There should be no shame because the 1st man and woman had sex in a park or garden and their kids also had sex outside, so if you and your partner afraid to have sex in public, it's most likely your relationship is limited and isn't that strong yet.*

LIST OF SEXUAL HERBS

If your sexual moods are suspended here's a list herbs that can improve your sex drive and promote sexual health. Some of these herbs are recognized as aphrodisiacs. I've selected the friendliest herbs that are easy to find in a health food store or herb shop. To be safe, only use these herbs after consulting with a physician, especially if you are diabetic or have a heart condition.

1. **Damiana**-This is a small green shrub with yellow flowers that is found throughout Mexico and South America. Indigenous people of the region have long used Damiana as an aphrodisiac, it's ideal in tea, and I recommend adding a sweet herb to it such as peppermint or spearmint, since Damiana has a slightly bitter taste. Women who drink a cup of Damiana tea one or two hours before having sex experience heightened

pleasure. Don't take Damiana if you are diabetic.

2. **Gingko Biloba**-Also known as the maiden hair tree, this herb has been shown to increase circulation in blood vessels just below the surface without increasing blood pressure. So its ideal to use for erectile difficulties. 3. **Yohimbe**-This African herb has been shown to improve a man's staying power. You need to wait about 30 minutes for Yohimbe to take effect. And the effect last for several hours. Take safety measures when using Yohimbe and use it responsibly and talk to your doctor first. If you have high blood pressure or diabetes, use Yohimbe only under the care of a doctor. Also don't take it with diet aids, commercial nasal decongestants that contain ephedrine, or with cheese, red wine or liver, since combining any of these, Yohimbine sometimes causes side effects including headaches. 4. **L-Arginine**-This non-essential amino acid is used in

sexual stimulants, since people who has used it report longer and more intense orgasms. In men, L-Arginine improves blood flow, resulting in harder, bigger and longer lasting erections. In women, L-Arginine encourages blood flow to the vaginal area making the vaginal tissues and clitoris more sensitive and very responsive to sexual stimulation. Women who increase their L-Arginine intake are better able to reach orgasm. 5. **Saw Palmetto**-This herb has long been recognized for its healing properties regarding the prostate gland in men. It also helps to alleviate hair loss in both men and women. This herb has an interesting effect on women regarding their hair because it both alleviates hair loss in women as well as reduces excessive grow of dark facial hair. Saw Palmetto has been prescribed for women suffering from acne and irregular menstrual cycles. It has also been used by women to enhance milk production in new mothers, increase breast size, and decrease menopausal problems. Do not take Saw Palmetto when pregnant, nursing, or trying to conceive. 6. **Ginseng**-Long revered for its sexual properties, Ginseng promotes blood production and encourages the secretion of sex hormones in men and women. Ginseng strengthens a man's sex organs. It also boosts sexuality, circulation, and energy. Ginseng improves your vitality and generally energy. So it's good to take for overall health reasons whether you are male or female. 7. **Sarsaparilla**-The root of this vitamin and mineral packed vine aids both men and women in the production of sex hormones testosterone, progesterone, and desoxy-corticosterone, saponins and plant steroids found in many species such as estrogen and testosterone. Please do not confuse this plant with the sarsaparilla that is used to flavor tasty soft drinks. 8. **Ginger**-This tasty root (not the powered spice variety) has been deemed an aphrodisiac for centuries because of its heady smell and the way in which it promotes circulation. Fresh ginger root steeped in tea also eases stomach pain. 9. **Avena Sativa (wild oats)**-Avena Sativa, or oats, have long been used by breeders to help mate animals "sow their oats" or boost their fertility. Avena Sativa is one of the best remedies to feed the nervous system when under stress and strengthen it to handle the situation. It works to calm down performance anxiety. 10. **Horny Goat Weed**-(epimedium) This Chinese herb is also known as Goat Sex Herb. It has been used for centuries to improve sexual functions. It has Androgen-like effects. Androgens are involved in sexual desire in both men and women. Horny Goat Weed may help improve circulation and kidney function. 11. **Maca Root**-

Grown high in the mountains of Peru, Maca Root tends to significantly boost libido sex drive in men and women by enhancing the endocrine function. The endocrine system includes all of the glands, and the hormones they secrete, function, digestion, brain and nervous system physiology, and energy levels. 12. **Brazilian Catoba bark**-Brazil's most famous and highly regarded libido booster. It is considered a central nervous system stimulant and used for sexual weaknesses and lowered libido in both men and women. 13. **Longifolia Jack**- (Tongkatali) A popular Malaysian tree, it is proper for its aphrodisiac properties for both men and women. The researched focus is towards improved desire and sexual iniation. 14. **Muira Pauma**-Found in Amazon, this extraction is very potent and has an impressive research history of helping restore libido and has been used to help prevent Erectile Dysfunction. 15.

Mucana Pruriens Extract-A rare and powerful Ayurvedic herb that has unusually high levels of naturally occurring L-Dopail. L-Dopa is an amino acid that has been subject of over 25 years of extensive scientific and medical research. It may help with improving sexual dysfunction, loss of libido, stimulating arousal, and increasing intensity and frequency of orgasms for both men and women. 16. **Tribulu Terrestnis**-Also known as puncture vine and Gokshura, may help to increase seminal fluid, not by volume but sperm count, and at the same time may increase sexual desire, arousal and performance in men and women. Tribulus may help to increase the duration of erection and assist in achieving orgasm in those previously unable.

SEX POSITIONS

69- Simultaneous oral sex between two people is called 69. They can be lying sided by side, lying one on top of the other or standing with one partner holding the other upside down.

T-Square position- The female lies on her back with knees up and legs apart. The male lies on his side perpendicular to the receiver with the female hips under the arch formed by her legs.

Knee Pile Driver- Start this inverted delight by lying flat on the ground face up. With your hands supporting your back, lift your legs and back side way, way up so they're as perpendicular to the ground as you can get them. Have your man kneel before you, grab your ankles, and bring his knees to your shoulders. Then take his hands and ask him to hold your hip that will steady you both.

Hold his thighs for leverage and adjust so your genitals can join for some upside down action.

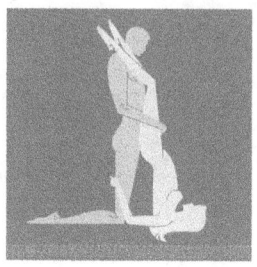

1 knee pile driver

Rated X- Have your man lie face up on the bed. Turn around and straddle him so your back is toward him, then lower yourself onto his penis. Extend your legs back toward his shoulders, relaxing your torso onto the bed between his feet. With both your legs and your man's forming an X-shape, start to slide up and down, use his feet for added pumping leverage. When the man decides to sit up then it's called the "bootyful view"

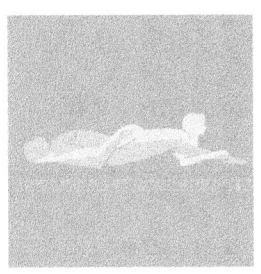

2 Rated X

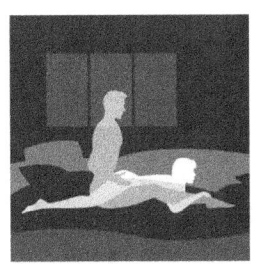

3 Rated X

Counter V- Sit on a counter and have him stand facing you. His legs should be slightly bent, spaced 3 feet apart with your arms on his shoulders and his arms around your lower back, slowly pull your right leg up and prop your right foot on his left shoulder. Then pull your left leg up and prop your left foot on his right shoulder.

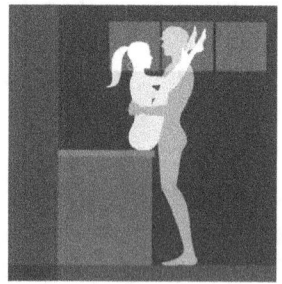

4 Counter V

Lotus- Get in lotus position with his legs crossed and each of his heels atop the opposite knee. Facing him sit in his lap and mount him with your legs wrapped snuggly around his waist.

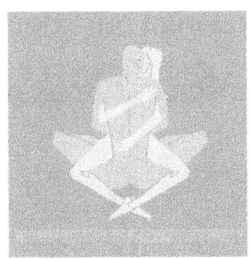

5 Lotus

Straddle Paddle- Sit your man down with your legs crossed. Facing him, straddle his legs and lower yourself into his lap without him penetrating you. Wrap your legs around either side of his torso, so they're hugging his buttocks. Then as you hold each other's arms or lower backs tightly, he enters you. Start slowly and rock back and forth together, increasing your speed as you come closer to climaxing

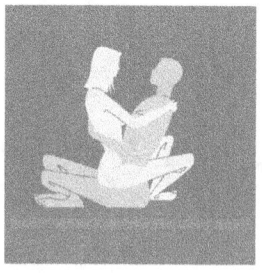

6Straddle Paddle

Real Lap Dance- While he's sitting in a low chair with his legs relaxed, straddle him with your feet on the floor, slowly lowering yourself onto him with your knees bent at a 90 degree angle. Start by letting just the tip of his penis enters you, then lower yourself inch by inch until all of him is inside you.

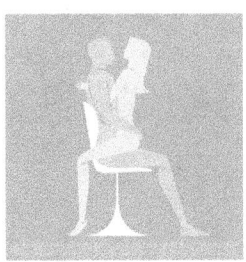

7 Real Lap Dance

Orgasmic- Find a chair and pad it with some pillows, straddle him and lean back slightly, placing your hands on his knees. Extend your legs until your ankles are resting on his shoulders. And then rock back and forth.

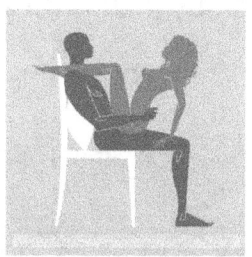

8 Orgasmic

Dream Come True- Your man lies on his back, his legs straight out in front of him and you straddle him with your head facing his feet, and you back up onto his penis while you thrusting, he holds your thighs or butt.

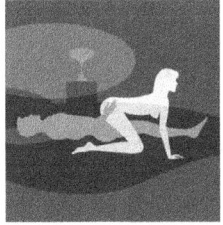

9 Dream Come True

The Erotic End- Sit your lover on the bed or floor with his legs stretched out in front of him. He leans back slightly using his arms to support his weight. With your back to him and your legs straddling his thighs, lower yourself onto him. Keep your knees bent and your feet planted on the floor. With your groins grinding together, squeeze your PC muscles while he makes small circular rotations on his pelvis.

Love Seat- The man lies back with his legs spread slightly, while she face the same direction with her back to his face, lowering herself onto his penis. Put your feet between his legs on the bed. Use your hands and your feet to thrust up and down on his penis.

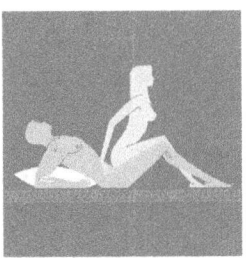

10 Love Seat

Thigh Coaster- The man lies on his back, one leg stretched and the other bent, knee pointing upward. She straddles him sideways with her back turned to his face and her stomach almost touching his bent knee. Use it for support as you rock back and forth or up and down.

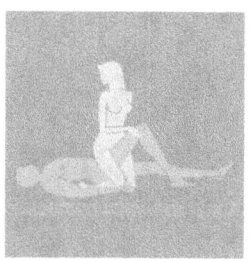

11 Thigh Coaster

Joy Ride- Your man lies on the bed on his back with his arms relaxed above his head. Straddle him on top and slide your legs straight out and forward, so that your feet are on either side of his shoulders. Hold his shins or push on the floor for leverage, and start moving your hips in figure 8 motions so you're moving his penis around like a joystick.

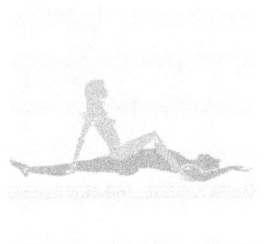

12 Joy Ride

Women Rules the World- He lying flat on his back with his knees bent and his legs spread apart. Get on top and slowly lower yourself onto his thing, keeping your knees bent and your legs outside his arms. Then lean back and support yourself on your palms as he moves his hips up and down.

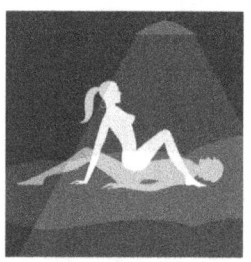

13 Women Rules the World

Up Up away- Standing with his back against the edge of the bed, he picks you up with his hands gripping your bottom and the backs of your thighs. Wrap your legs around his waist, place your feet on the bed for support and your arms around his neck and shoulders. As he enters, you hang motion up and down with the help of his arms.

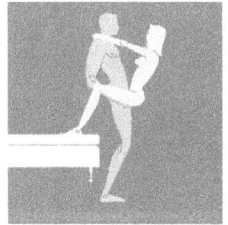

14 Up Up Away

Bed Shaker Doggy style- lie face down on a bed with your feet flat on the floor, while he enters from behind.

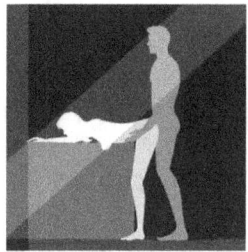

15 Bed Shaker Doggy style

Love Couch- Have your partner sit back on a couch. Straddle his lap with your legs apart and your knees bent up against his chest. Then lean back so you're almost upside down with your arms stretched behind you.

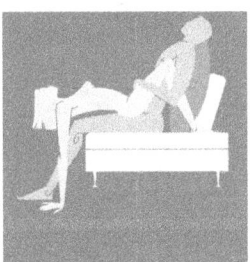

16 Love Couch

Straight Doggy- While standing up, bend forward with your legs spread slightly, keep your back straight and your hands resting on your knees for balance, he enters from behind pulling himself close to you while holding onto your waist for support.

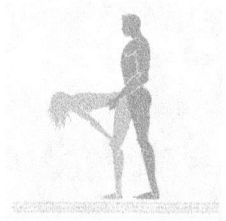

17 Straight Doggy

All Up In It- Lie down on your stomach and keeping your legs straight spread them slightly. Rest your arms by your side or stretch them out in front of you. Have him stretch his body over yours, resting on his elbows so he doesn't place all his weight on you. He then positions his legs outside your legs. As he enters you, close your legs and cross them at the ankles.

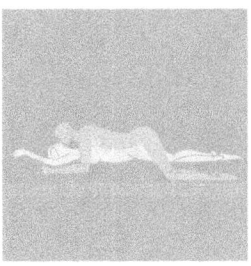

18 All Up In It

Doggy Off The Edge- Pose on all fours with your knees at the edge of the bed while he stands behind you, his feet hip width apart. While he spreads his legs on either side of yours, keep your knees together to narrow your vaginal canal, causing it to feel much snugger around his penis as he thrusts.

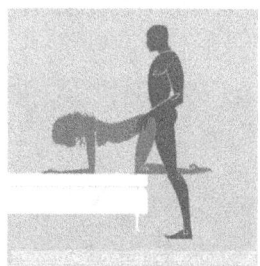

19 Doggy Off The Edge

Ballerina- Face your partner, standing with your legs shoulder width apart. Take your left foot and turn it out to the side while keeping your right one facing forward. Wrap your arms around his neck; pull your right leg up and over his shoulder. Keeping your right knee bent as he slowly enters you.

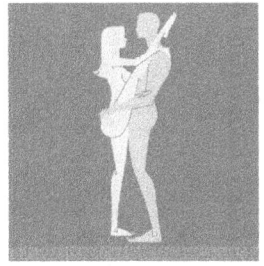

20 Ballerina

The Doctor Cure- Lie face-up at the edge of the bed. Place a pillow under your butt to get some elevation. Extend your legs straight up. Keeping them close together, your man enters your vagina while standing up.

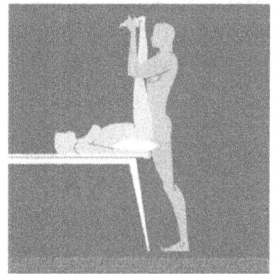

21 The Doctor's Cure

The Spider Web- Both you and your partner lie on your sides facing each other. Lean in close together and scissor your legs through his so you're super close and he's deep inside you as he enters you. While thrusting, hold on to each other for leverage and ultimate friction.

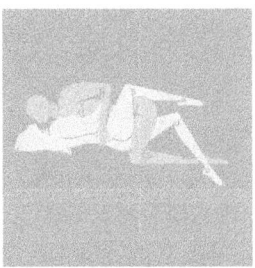

22 The Spider Web

Open Wide- Lie on your side with your guy behind you. Keep both of your torsos in this dose pose and lift your top leg. Have him shift his lower body into half-kneeing position, entering you from behind. This is the half doggy style.

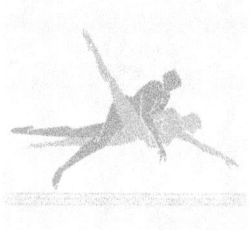

23 Open Wide

The Fantasy- You lie on your side on the bed or floor, turned away from your guy with your legs straight out in front of you at a ninety degree angle to your torso. Your guy lies behind you on his side in a modified position, lines up his genitals with yours, then raises his torso with his arms, entering you he controls the motion as he moves in and out.

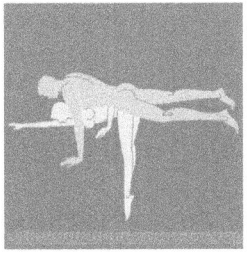

24 The Fantasy

List of STDs (Sexually Transmitted Disease)

Facts STDs (Sexually Transmitted Disease) Preventions

STDs aka STIs, is definitely something to think about. But if you get the right information and get tested, you can put an end to the guessing game and stay confident. There's a list of STDs for all facts. And remember, if you test positive for any STI, you should inform all recent sexual partners (past 60 days) so they can get tested and treated too. Here in this chapter is a list of all common STDs that sneak up on human lives every day.

1. BACTERIAL VAGINOSIS (BV)

2. CHALAMYDIA

3. GONORRHEA

4. HERPES

5. HUMAN PAILLOMAVIRUS (HPV & GENITAL WARTS

6. TRICHOMONIASIS

7. CHANROID

8. HEPATITIS

9. HIV/AIDS

10. LYMPHOGRANULOMAVENEREAM (LVG)

11. MOLLUSCUM CONTAGIOSUM

12. MUCOPURULENT LERUICILIS (MPC)

13. PELVIC INFLAMMATORY DISEASE (PID)

14. PUBIC "CRAB" LICE

15. SCABIES

16. SYPHILIS

BACTERIAL VAGINOSIS (BV)

BV is a vaginal infection caused by an imbalance of bacteria. It can be spread through both sexual and non-sexual contact. BV is the most common vaginal infection in women of reproductive age and it occurs when there is an overgrowth of certain "bad" bacterial in the vaginal. BV occurs when the balance between "good" and "harmful" bacterial is thrown off. Often there are no symptoms at all, but sometimes BV is accompanied by unusual discharge, strong odor, painful urination, itching, or burning. BV can be treated with antibiotic pills, vaginal creams or suppositors. Sometimes BV will clear up on its own, but getting treatment is important to avoid complications. BV is considered a sexual associated infection, not specifically an STI. This is because it can be spread through sexual contact, but women can also get this infection unrelated to sexual activity. It is simply an imbalance in the bacterial in the vagina. Keeping the vagina clean, using condoms or stay monogamous with a long term partner can help reduce the risk or/and prevent BV from occurring. Also avoid douching, as this can remove good bacteria and make BV worse. A health care provider will examine the vagina for signs of BV and take a sample of vagina fluid to be examined under a microscope or sent to a lab for testing. Schedule the test when you are not on your period. Do not have sex, douche or use a tampon within 24 hours of your exam.

CHLAMDIA

Chlamydia is the number one cause of preventable infertility in the US. CHLAMYDIA is one of the most common STDs and the leading cause of preventable infertility in the United States. If left untreated, CHLAMYDIA may also lead to pelvic inflammatory disease and the risk of ectopic pregnancy in women. CHLAMYDIA is both treatable and preventable. Most people with CHLAMYDIA don't have any symptoms, but those who do might have unusual genital discharge and/or pain and burning urinating. Women may also have lower back or abdominal pain, nausea, pain during sex, or bleeding after sex or between periods. CHLAMYDIA is treated with antibiotics; some antibiotics can cure it in just one dose, while others may need to be used for several days. If you been treated, your partner should get tested or treated too. And you should wait seven days or until you and your partner finish the antibiotics before having sex again, to make sure you don't spread the disease. CHLAMYDIA can be spread by oral, anal or vaginal sex and cause infection in the anus, mouth or throat in penis or vagina. The most effective protection is to be monogamous with a long term partner who tested negative for CHLAMYDIA, using latex condoms or dental dams can also help reduce the risk of contracting or spreading the infection. A urine test is the easiest way to detect CHLAMYDIA, but women have a couple of other options. You can also have your doctor do a cervical swab test, or you can do a vaginal swab. Caused by the bacterium, CHLAMYDIA TRACHOMATIS, which can damage a woman's reproductive organs. CHLAMYDIA can cause discharge from the penis of an infected man. The greater the number of sex partners, the greater the risk. Since CHLAMYDIA can be transmitted by oral and anal sex, men who have sex with men are at greater risk.

GONORRHEA

The rate of 15-29 year old Coloradoans with GONORRHEA is twice the overall national rate. GONORRHEA is one of the most common STDs in the United States and can lead to infertility in men and women. It is both treatable and preventable, though scientists have discovered a new strain of GONORRHEA that is resistant to all currently utilized antibiotics. Many people with GONORRHEA don't have any symptoms. Those who do might notice unusual discharge from the penis or vagina and/or pain or difficult peeing. Men may have swelling in their testicles and women may bleed in between periods. If left untreated, GONORRHEA can cause infertility without ever showing symptoms. It can also spread to the blood and joints. GONORRHEA is treated with antibiotics, usually given in a single dose. If you're being treated, your partner should be tested too. You should also wait until you and your partner finish your treatment and until your symptoms disappear before you start having sex again; to make sure you don't spread the infection. In addition to the urethra and vagina, GONORRHEA can also cause infections in the mouth, throat, eyes and anus. The most effective protection is using condoms or staying monogamous with one long term partner who has tested negative for GONORRHEA.

Other Info: GONORRHEA is a sexually transmitted disease caused by a bacterium. It can grow easily in the warm, moist areas of the reproductive tract, including the cervix opening to the womb, uterus (womb) and fallopian tubes (egg canals) in women, and in the urethra (urine canal) in women and men. The bacterium can also grow in the mouth, throat, eyes and anus. People get GONORRHEA by having sex with someone who has the disease. GONORRHEA can be transmitted via fluids even if a man does not ejaculate. It can also be spread from an untreated mother to her baby during child birth. Untreated GONORRHEA can cause serious and permanent health problems in both women and men. Untreated GONORRHEA can increase a person's risk of acquiring or transmitting HIV-the virus that causes AIDS. TO test GONORRHEA, usually you'll do a urine test, but some health care providers will use a swab to collect a sample.

HERPES

There is no cure for herpes, but certain meds can shorten and prevent outbreaks when taken regularly. HERPES is a common STD and a lot of people who have it don't even know. There is no cure for HERPES, but there is a treatment that can lessen symptoms and decrease the chance of passing it on to someone else. Most of the time HERPES doesn't cause any symptoms when there are signs and they can include blisters around the genital, or anus. The first outbreak of sores is usually the worst. A person with HERPES may have additional outbreaks of sores weeks or months after the first outbreak. These additional outbreaks are less severe, heal faster and occur less often overtime, condoms can help reduce the risk of passing HERPES from one person to another, but they are not 100% effective. If you or your partner is having an outbreak of sores, you should abstain until they are fully healed. It is much easier to pass or catch the virus when sores are present. The most effective prevention is staying monogamous with a long term partner who has been tested negative for herpes. But because herpes is spread through skin to skin contact, condoms do not fully protect against the spread of the virus. If you have an outbreak of sores, a doctor can usually diagnose HERPES by looking at the sores; to be sure, he can also take a swab sample and test it in the lab. Or a blood test can be taken. People get HERPES by having sex with someone who has the disease (oral, anus or vagina sex). Genital HERPES can cause painful genital sores in many adults and can be severe in people with suppressed immune systems. If a person with genital HERPES touches their sores or the fluids from the sores, they may transfer HERPES to another part of the body. If they are touch, immediate and thorough hand washing make the transfer less likely. Genital HERPES can cause sores or breaks in the skin or Mucous membranes (lining of the mouth, vagina, and rectum). The genital sores caused by HERPES can easily bleed. When the sores come into contact with the mouth, vagina or rectum during sex, they increase the risk of HIV transmission if either partner is HIV infected.

HUMAN PAILLOMAVIRS (HPV) AND GENITAL WARTS

HPV is the most common STD and at less 50% of sexually active people will get it at some time in their lives. The body usually clears HPV on its own without causing problems, but HPV can lead to certain kinds of cancer. There are more than 100 different kinds of HPV. Most of the time there are no symptoms and the virus clears on its own, but several types can cause genital warts or lead to vaginal, anal, throat, and cervical cancer. The types of HPV that causes warts do not cause cancer, but they can indicate a higher risk for having the types of HPV that are linked to cancer. They types of HPV that cause cancer do not show any signs. Treatment: The body will usually clear HPV infections on its own within a couple of months. Warts can be treated in several different ways. Creams, gels and solutions, or you can freeze them off with liquid nitrogen, or you can burn them off with trichloroacetic acid or bichluracetic acid; or simply apply a tincture or ointment that will remove the warts. A doctor can cut off the warts using scalpel, scissors, curette or electro-surgery. Cancer causing HPV can be monitored in females through regular Pap tests, but there is no specific treatment to eliminate HPV from the body. If the HPV causes abnormal cells to form, a doctor will likely remove the cells and biopsy them. Depending on the types of abnormalities, the doctor may recommend a colposcopy a special exam that magnifies the walls of the vagina and cervix) or LEEP (a procedure to remove the abnormal cells before they can cause cancer). HPV is extremely common and there is no general test for the virus' many forms. Although there are no cures, the body will usually clear the HPV infection on its own. The most effective prevention is using latex condoms and staying monogamous with a long term partner who has been tested negative. Genital warts are typically diagnosed through a visual examination. Your doctor may apply a weak vinegar solution because the acidity will make the warts turn white and become more visible.

TRICHOMONIASIS

TRICHOMONIASIS is the most common curable STI. It can be treated with antibiotics; signs in women include excessive, frothy, yellowish or greenish vaginal discharge. There may also be swelling of the vulva and labia along with painful urination. Symptoms in men may include painful urination with lesions on the penis, but most men with TRICHOMONIASIS will have no symptoms. It is important to be treated because reinfection is very common. Avoid drinking alcohol until 24-48 hours after finishing treatment. TRICHOMONIASIS has been linked to an increased risk of HIV acquisition. Staying monogamous and using latex condoms can help reduce the spread of infection. Testing involves having a health care provider take a swab sample from the infected area to examine under a microscope or send to a lab. Also pregnant women with TRICHOMONIASIS can deliver premature, low birth weight babies.

CHANROID

Is a bacteria STI that causes painful ulcers or sores in the genital region. Women with CHANROID often have no symptoms. Men will usually have a painful, erosive ulcer with ragged edges somewhere on the penis. Tissue around the sores can die and lead to more serious infection if not treated. CHANROID is not very common in the United States and is most often seen among commercial sex workers or their sex partners. The most effective solution is to be monogamous with a long term partner and using latex condoms. In order to diagnose CHANROID, a health care provider will examine the ulcer using a special type of microscope, or a sample can be taken and cultured.

HEPATITIS

There are several kinds of HEPATITIS, but HEPATITIS B is the one most likely to be transmitted sexually. There are three different kinds of HEPATITIS, some of which are spread more easily than others. HEPATITIS A, B and C can all be transmitted sexually; however HEPATITIS B is the type most likely to be sexually transmitted. All types of HEPATITIS are serious and affect the liver. HEPATITIS B and C are the leading cause of liver cancer and are the most common reason for liver transplants. Most HAV infections will cause symptoms including fatigue, loss of appetite, nausea, vomiting, headache, fever, dark urine, jaundice and liver enlargement and tenderness. There are no specific cures for HAV or HBV. There are treatments that can lessen the symptoms. HAV is spread through fecal contamination, meaning that it can be spread through anal sex. HAV can also be spread by people preparing or eating food after going to the bathroom and not washing their hands.

HIV/AIDS

The human Immune deficiency Virus (HIV) is the virus that causes Acquired Immune Deficiency syndrome (AIDS) is transmitted by blood and body fluids. Most HIV infections do not have any symptoms. A person infected with HIV can remain healthy and symptom-free for many years. If HIV leads to AIDS, serious symptoms can develop and can ultimately lead to death. Signs and symptoms may include everything from fever and rashes to lesions, soaking night sweats and blurred vision. There is no cure for HIV, but there are treatment options that allow HIV-positive individuals to live long, healthy lives. If someone is exposed to HIV, or think he or she may have been exposed, there is a post-exposure prophylatis (PEP) that can reduce the chance of HIV infection occurring. PEP is medication that should be started as quickly as possible, no later than 72 hours after the exposure. Although treatment options have improved greatly in recent years. HIV remains a very serious threat. Many people are unaware of their status until later stages, but unfortunately people are the most contagious soon after becoming infected. Being infected with other STIs can make you more susceptible to HIV. The most effective prevention is staying monogamous with a long term partner who has been tested negative for HIV. Latex condoms can help reduce the risk of contracting or spreading the infection. In addition to sex, HIV can be transmitted through any one of the following: the process of delivering a baby, breast feeding if the mother is infected, and sharing needles. There are a couple of different tests for HIV. The best option is blood test. A rapid test can also be done using either blood or a swab from the inside of the cheek. Usually, if the initial test is positive, it will be followed up with a more sensitive blood test to confirm the results. Rapid tests take about 15-20 minutes, while a blood test sent to the lab will take up to a week to get virus. If HIV is contracted, it can take three weeks to up to six months for any test to detect HIV.

LYMPHOGRANULOMA VENEREUM (LGV)

LGV is fairly uncommon and is most often spread through unprotected anal sex. The first sign of LGV is a small painless ulcer at the point of infection- it may be so small, in fact, that it goes unnoticed. Swollen lymph nodes are the most common sign and usually appear a week to month later. Stiffness and aching in the groin may also occur. LGV can be treated with a 3-week course of antibiotics. If you or your partner is diagnosed with LGV, you should abstain from sex until your treatment is complete and all symptoms disappear to avoid reinfection. The best way to prevent LGV is to avoid anal sex. LGV can be difficult to diagnose because many of the symptoms are similar to other infections. Most diagnoses are made based on health center observations, but samples can be taken from lesions or sores and tested for the bacteria.

MOLLUSCUM CONTAGIOSUM

MOLLUSCUM CONTAGIOSUM is caused by a virus that can be spread sexually and by no-sexual contact through contaminated objects like towels, clothing or sex toys. Symptoms include shiny smooth white dimpled bumps with a curd-like core and itching on the genitals and trunk area. MOLLUSCUM CONTAGLOSUM will usually go away on its own within a year without treatment. The bumps can be removed by a doctor in a number of different ways, which is usually done only when there are ten or fewer lesions. Sometimes MOLLUSCUM CONTAGLOSUM can lead to a more serious infection such as staphylococcus, so lesions should be monitored for signs of infection. The best prevention is to wash your hands daily, use clean towels, face rags, and use latex condoms. MOLLUSCUM CONTAGLOSUM is diagnosed based on visual examination. Samples of the bumps may be examined under a microscope to detect the virus.

MUCOPURULENT CERVICITIS (MPC)

MPC is caused by other STDs such as CHLAMYDIA or GONORRHEA and maybe treatable with antibiotics, it can lead to PID if left untreated. Although MPC sometimes comes with no signs or symptoms, for women it can cause bleeding during or after sex. unusual vaginal discharge, spotting between periods, lower abdominal pain or pain during sex. Depending on symptoms and the results of other STI tests, there are several different kinds of antibiotics that might be prescribed to treat MPC. Even after treatment, you may be asked to schedule a follow-up to make sure the infection is totally cleared up and there is no risk of getting PID later. Avoid douching because it can actually hide the symptoms of MPC, making it harder to diagnose and treat. Best prevention is staying monogamous with a long term partner and using latex condoms. There is no specific test for MPC, but a health care provider can diagnose the infection based on symptoms and a visual examination of a patients genitals. The provider will look for white blood cells or pus, which may indicate MPC. Because MPC can be caused by other STIs, a health care provider will probably test for CHLAMYDIA, GONORRHEA or other infections based on a patient's sexual history of symptoms.

PELVIC INFLAMMATORY DISEASE (PID)

PID is caused by bacteria, which often stem from another STD such as CHLAMYDIA or GONORRHEA. It occurs when these bacterial move up from vagina or cervix into the uterus and other reproductive organs. Many women with PID don't have any symptoms at all. If they do have symptoms, they may include abdominal, cervical or uterine pain or tenderness, along with fever or chills. Symptoms of PID usually occur in the first five to ten days of a woman's menstrual cycle. Numerous bacteria can cause PID, so it is treated with a combination of antibiotics. Depending on the severity of symptoms, antibiotics may be given through an IV or orally. Some PID infections may require hospitalization. If left untreated, PID can have potentially life threatening complications, including ectopic pregnancy and pelvic abscess. It can also lead to infertility, chronic abdominal pain, pelvic scar tissue, premature hysterectomy and depression. Best prevention is to stay monogamous with a long term partner and use latex condoms. Diagnose is usually based on the presence of typical symptoms when other serious conditions like appendicitis or ectopic pregnancy can be excluded. In rare, cases, a health care provider may use a laparoscope to view the fallopian tubes to confirm inflammations. Appropriate treatment of PID can help prevent complications, including permanent damage to female reproductive organs.

PUBIC "CRAB" LICE

Pubic lice are parasites that can cause itching, blue spots and sores in the infected area. "Crabs" are parasitic insects that survive by feeding on human blood. Pubic lice are different parasites than head or body lice and are usually found in the pubic hair, but can also be found in other course body hair like eyebrows, beard, chest or armpit hair. "Crabs" the symptoms would help you be able to see grey-white lice or hair nits (the egg form of pubic lice). Prescription or over the counter shampoos or solutions can be used to treat "Crab" pubic lice. In addition to treating the lice. Clothing and bedding should be washed in hot water and dried in a dryer or dry cleaned. It is not necessary to fumigate living quarters. Although pubic "Crabs" lice are most commonly spread through sexual contact, they can be spread through sharing clothing or bedding with someone who has pubic lice. They are not spread by cats, dogs, or other animals. The most effective prevention is to be monogamous with a long term partner or to use latex condoms. The test for pubic "Crab" lice is a visual examination. Your health care provider will usually remove hair or a few hairs with nits to examine under a microscope.

SCABIES

SCABIES are parasites that infect the skin. They can be passed just through skin to skin contact of any kind, sexual or not. It can cause intense itching and pimply rash. The itching will often be worse at night than during the day. Itching and a rash most often show up on the penis, buttocks, wrist, nipples, waist, shoulder blades, armpits, elbows and between the fingers, but it is not limited to these areas. Sometimes SCABIES might also result in tiny burrows in the skin caused by the female mites tunneling beneath the skin. If a person has SCABIES for the first time, it will usually take 2-4 weeks for symptoms to start appearing. For those who have had SCABIES before, symptoms can occur in as little as 24 hours. It is important to know that even when symptoms are not present, SCABIES can still spread. Prescription creams called Scabicides can be used to treat SCABIES. These creams kill the mites and some also kill the eggs. The cream will be applied to the skin from the neck down to the toes and washed off after 8-14 hours. There is also an antibiotic that can be taken by mouth in a single dose, followed by another single dose two weeks later. Because SCABIES are so easy to pass from one person to another, any sexual partners and close personal or house hold contacts should be examined and treated. Bedding and clothing must also be decontaminated by machine washing and drying on hot cycle or day cleaning. Removing from body contract for at least 72 hours will also ensure that the mites can't be transmitted. Although SCABIES is most commonly spread through skin to skin contact, it can be spread through sexual contact with someone who has SCABIES. The best effective prevention is to be monogamous with a long term partner and use latex condoms. The test for SCABIES is a visual examination, most of the time; a diagnosis can be made based on history of exposure to SCABIES or the presence of common symptoms like rash and itching that gets worse at night. A health care provider might also take a scraping of this infected skin to examine under a microscope to look for mites eggs, larvae, or feces.

SYPHILIS

SYPHILIS is spread by contact with open sores usually during sex. If left untreated it can cause serious health problems, including brain and nervous system damage, blood infection and even death. If early action is taken, SYPHILIS can be cured with antibiotics. SYPHILIS prevalence is growing in the United States. Particularly among men who have sex with men. Early signs may include a small, painless, firm sore in or around the vagina, penis, mouth, or anus. This can be followed by rash on the body that is particularly noticeable on the palms of the hands or sores of the feet. Other, less common signs and symptoms may include fever, swollen lymph glands, sore throat, patchy hair loss, headaches, weight loss, muscle aches, and fatigue. Early-diagnosed syphilis can be treated and cured easily with an injection of penicillin or 14 days of antibiotics for patients allergic to penicillin. For people who have syphilis that was undiagnosed for more than one year, it can be treated and cured with a longer course of stronger antibiotics (an injection once a week for three weeks). If pregnant women contracts SYPHILIS, it can lead to the death of the fetus. SYPHILIS can be spread through oral, vagina, and anal sex with sores being present on the lips, mouth and anus in addition to the genitals. The most effective prevention is to be monogamous with one long term partner and to use latex condoms. The test used for diagnosis will depend on what symptoms are present and how much time has passed since exposure. SYPHILIS can be diagnosed by blood test, or by examining a sample from a sore. If no symptoms are present, these tests may not be able to identify a SYPHILIS infection.

67% of all SYPHILIS occurred among men who have sex with men. There were also 377 reports of children with congenital SYPHILIS. Oral, Anal, Vaginal or Penile SYPHILIS sores make it easier to transmit and acquire HIV infection. A person is 2 to 5 times more likely to get HIV if exposed when SYPHILIS sores are present.

www.ingramcontent.com/pod-product-compliance
Lightning Source LLC
Chambersburg PA
CBHW070559290526
45790CB00002B/734